Yoga For Better Vision Health

Improve Your Eye Sight With Yoga Practice

By

ASHIA Gill

Table of Contents

Summary

Eye tiredness affects not just the eyes, but also the neck and the back of the head. My body and eyes have been stressed for a long time because I don't know how to properly rest them. You need to let your body and eyes relax, give yourself time to be confused, and give yourself time to move. Eye problems are often caused by things that people do every day.

What is Eye Yoga

Because people spend so much time in front of screens on phones, TVs, tablets, and computers, their eyes are put through a lot of stress every day. This makes the lenses, muscles, and ocular receptors work harder than they should, which makes them tired and can cause more or less major problems. To try to get rid of them, Eye Yoga could be helpful. It's a way to relax that uses specific moves to strengthen the muscles, give you instant relief, and give you other benefits.

Facial gymnastics can also be done to keep the eyes and the area around them healthy and to avoid getting crow's feet.

How does it work

Depending on the exercise, the method usually involves looking at something close up or far away for a few seconds and then moving your eyes in a certain way to the left, right, up, or down.

What is the mind-body connection

The mind-body relationship is the link between how a person thinks, feels, and acts and how healthy their body is.

Scientists have known for a long time that our feelings can change how our bodies work, but we're just now starting to learn how emotions affect our health and how long we live.

Holistic medicine is a type of health care that tries to help the whole person, not just their symptoms. One important part of holistic medicine is the mind-body connection. Now more than ever, doctors know how important it is to treat the whole person, including their mind, body, and spirit.

How yoga and meditation are good for the body and brain

How yoga and meditation are good for the body and brain

Mind, body, and spirit are all connected, and yoga and meditation help us learn more about this. Studies have shown that the vagus nerve is involved in the relaxation reaction, which is also called the "rest-and-digest" system. So, yoga moves the nervous system out of the stress-related "fight, flight, or freeze" response and into the "rest and digest" response, which improves mental health.

Also, yoga raises the amount of GABA in the brain, which is a chemical that helps calm the mind. In a 12-week study, people walked for an hour three times a week or did yoga. The yoga group's GABA levels went up more, their mood improved more, and the physical affects of anxiety went down more.

The Link Between Eyes and Brain

The connection between the eyes and the mind is real, even if it seems like a fantasy. About 40% of the brain is used for vision, which is why we close our eyes to relax and fall asleep. And four of our 12 cranial nerves are only for seeing, while two others are also linked to seeing. Compare this to the heart and stomach systems, which are controlled by just one cranial nerve.

Even though the main goal of eye asanas may be to gain clarity, improving vision is also an important benefit. Surprisingly, it doesn't seem to be the stretching and tightening of muscles that helps the most. Relaxing seems to be the most important thing for healthy eyes. In a trial, when people put the muscle relaxant curare on their eyes, their vision got a lot better.

Alleged benefits

Even though there is no scientific proof that Eye Yoga movements can actually fix astigmatism, myopia, or hyperopia, strengthening the muscles of the eye structure can help people who have trouble seeing.

Some studies, though, say that they can help lower eye pressure, which could slow the development of glaucoma. Also, it would help the eye get stronger after surgery for cataracts.

This is why, if you wear contact lenses, you should always take them out at night.

Relieve stress

However, the movements of focusing and muscle training are useful for two purposes. First, they make you feel calm and relaxed, which can help ease stress and treat things like headaches, high blood pressure, and anxiety.

Second, doing Eye Yoga can help the brain better understand what the eyes are telling it. This doesn't mean that your eyesight actually gets better, but you may be able to pay more attention to what you see and feel like you can see better because of it.

This may be why a scientific study couldn't find a way to scientifically measure how much better people's vision got after doing Eye Yoga, but people who did it still felt better.

Fights eye fatigue

Yoga for the eyes can also help avoid and treat eyestrain. A study of 60 students shows that this is true. After 8 weeks of practise, they were less tired and their eyes didn't hurt as much.

Stress is linked to eyestrain, so this benefit can be measured by improving muscles and reducing stress, which helps you stay focused.

The benefits of yoga for eyesight

Eye yoga, here are the main benefits:

- reduces eye pressure;
- helps to strengthen eye strength;
- improves ability to focus;
- relaxes the eyes and consequently the sense of fatigue is significantly reduced;
- it helps to pay more attention to what you see, and therefore you have the sensation of seeing in a clearer and more centered way.

Yoga exercises for the eyes

Here we are at the central point of our article, with no less than six yoga exercises for the eyes .

Trataka

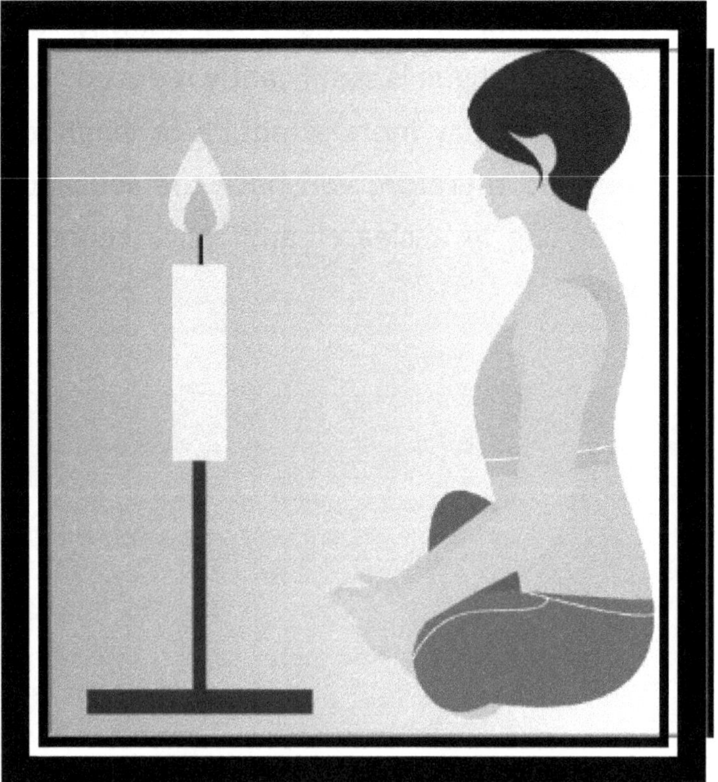

Set yourself up in front of a lit candle with your back straight and the light right in front of your eyes.

He looks at the centre of the light, and he may not blink once. Even the first few times, it's not easy, but give it a shot.

Even if your eyes are watering, keep going for five minutes. This is a sign that the tear ducts are being cleaned.

At the end of the time, close your eyes and open them again several times, and then close your eyes and take a few deep breaths.

Focus

- Sitting, back straight, staring at the tip of the index finger, bring your finger between the eyebrows.
- Hold the position and gaze for 3-4 breaths.
- Still looking at your index finger, bring it forward with your arm fully extended.
- After a few breaths, reposition your finger between your eyebrows again.
- After the sequence, repeat it starting and returning to the tip of the nose.

Focus on the go

- Sit up straight, gaze straight ahead.
- Extend your left arm as far as you can, thumb pointing up.
- Focus on the thumb.
- Slowly move your arm first to the right, as far as you can, and then to the left, always following the thumb with your eyes.Make sure you don't move your neck..
- Repeat several times.

Eye rotation

- The starting position of this yoga exercise for eyes is always the same: sitting with a straight back.
- Look at the ceiling, trying to stay focused as much as possible.
- Then roll your eyes to the right, then up, then to the left.
- Return your gaze to the ceiling.
- Back to looking ahead.
- Repeat the rotation in this direction several times, then move your eyes counterclockwise following the same principle.

Decentralization

- Extend both arms forward, with thumbs raised.
- Fixing the center of the two thumbs, open your arms out to the side, very, very slowly. Make sure your head doesn't move.
- Hold the position for 6-7 breaths, then return to the initial position, always following the movement with your eyes.

Vertical look

- Extend your right arm forward, pointing your index finger to the left.
- With your gaze fixed on the center of the finger, lift your arm. It is also important in this case not to move the head.
- Keep lifting it until it disappears from view.
- Hold the position for 3-4 breaths, then lower your finger back to eye level.
- Repeat everything, moving your finger down.

Eyes are tired regardless of age

Eye problems have changed a lot in the last few years. In the past, many people tried to find a fix for myopia, but now most people have eye strain.

There must be a lot of people who need eye drops because they have tired eyes or pain behind their eyes.

Eye tiredness affects not just the eyes, but also the neck and the back of the head. Everyone has eye pain, no matter how old they are.

The main thing that causes eye strain is staring at a computer or smartphone for a long time. Simply put, some of the muscles and nerves in your eyes are being used too much. When you look around the train, you can see that everyone is looking at their phones. No one is looking at the scenery outside the window or at how the clouds are changing shape.

Even when we're close to something, we rarely see it from a long way away. People over 40 can now have a condition called "smartphone presbyopia," which means they can see close up but not far away.

Also, I don't know how to rest my body properly, so my body and eyes are always tense. You need to let your body and eyes relax, give yourself time to be confused, and give yourself time to move. Eye problems are often caused by things that people do every day. With this in mind, I came up with "eye yoga" to help people with problems like asthenopia, dry eyes, myopia, hyperopia, and presbyopia.

"Eye yoga" is also becoming more popular in art schools and company workshops.

At the culture school, we put up an eye test chart in the classroom and ask the students to check their eyesight before and after eye yoga. Then, most people who started with 0.1 get to 0.3, and most people who started with 0.3 get to 0.5.

Before I did eye yoga, I could see about two or three things higher than I can now. Also, I often hear that even in eye yoga classes, signs that couldn't be seen on the way to class could be seen on the way home.

Eye yoga soothes the tight muscles and nerves around the eyes. This helps move blood and energy that have become stuck. As a result, eye fatigue is eased and the field of vision gets brighter and clearer.

Imagery is important in yoga

First of all, yoga is a way of thinking and moving that helps you get the most out of your body and life. Eye yoga is all about making the most of what your eyes can do.

Because of the bad ways we use our bodies and eyes, we can't show off our original skills. "Eye yoga" brings out our original skills and makes us stronger.

Eye yoga is more than just movements for your eyes and body. Integrating the body, heart, and mind is very important.

By combining the "Three Cs"—body, breath, and mind—and using the power of breath and mind together while moving the body, you will be able to use yourbody, flexibility, and agility faster than ever before. It becomes normal.

The "Eye-Lighting Method" described here sends fresh "qi" from the hands to the eyes, warms the area around the eyes, improves blood flow, gets rid of tiredness and waste quickly, and is the yoga breathing technique for cleansing. It is the way the law is used on the eye.

Qi is the life force of a person. If a person's life energy is in a bad state, they are "sick," and if it is in a good state, they are "genki."

Let's improve this qi by using the power of our minds and breaths. Place the middle of your palm over your eyes and take a slow breath in as you imagine clean energy coming from your palm.

Next, slowly let out your breath while picturing your tired eyes coming out of your mouth. The blood flow around your eyes will get better as you breathe in and out.

Also, it helps to relax your body and tell yourself with each breath that the stress is getting less and less. If you do it slowly and carefully, you should be able to stop your eyes from getting tired and see better. To move your mind, it's important to picture what you want. By doing this, the movements of the body, the breath, and the mind will all be in sync, which will increase the benefits of yoga.

How to do eye yoga

The "eye illumination method" works even if you do it while sitting in a chair, but you can relax your body and mind by doing it while lying on your back in a "relaxation pose" that calms your whole body. I think it's good because it helps me sleep better.

1. Rub your palms together to warm them. Make your palms look like a bowl.

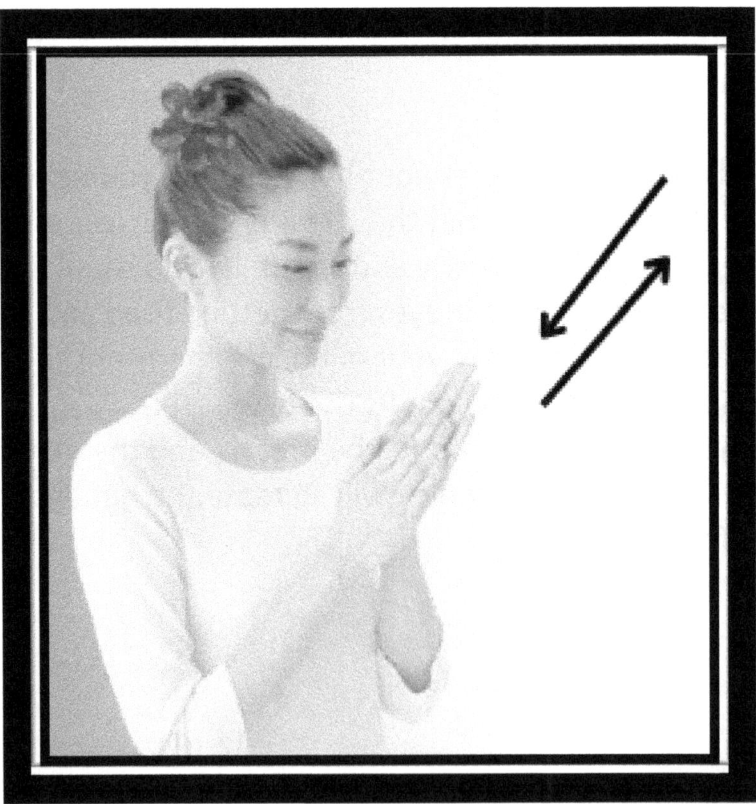

 Use both hands to cover both eyes. At this point, the palm's centre should be right above the eyes.

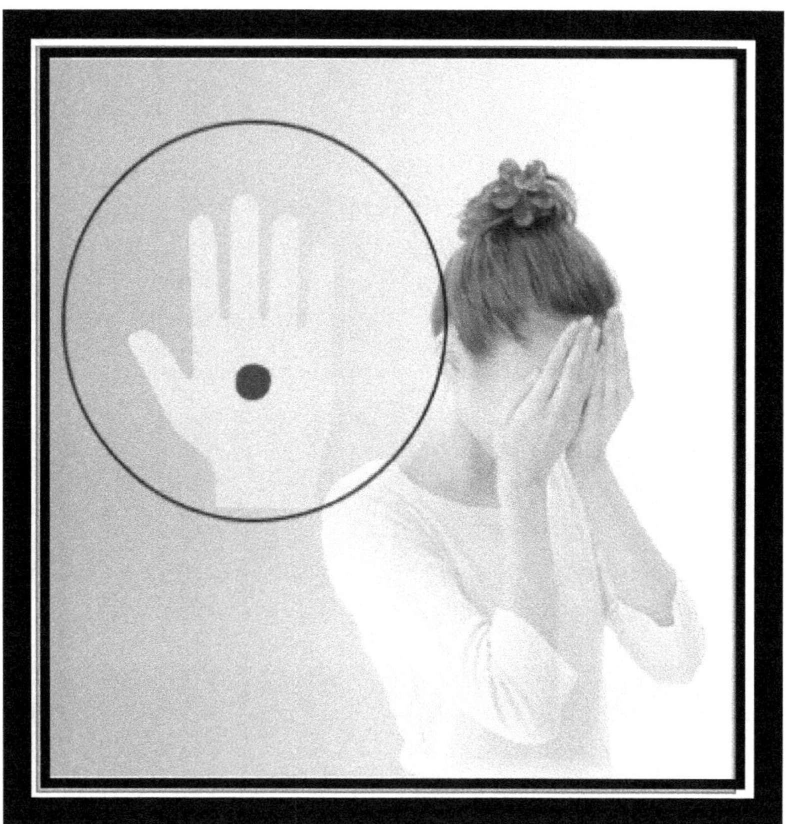

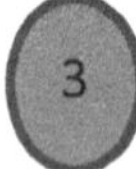

Imagine that you are taking in qi as you slowly inhale from the palm of your hand to your eyes.

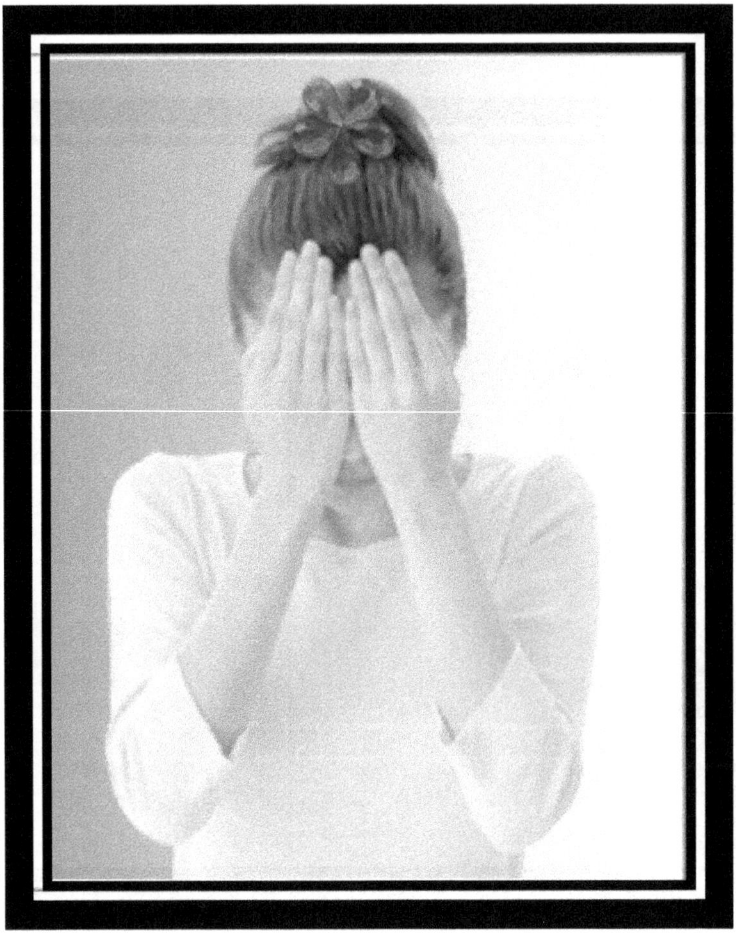

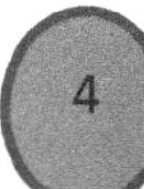

Slowly let your breath out through your mouth, as if you were letting out your tired eyes.

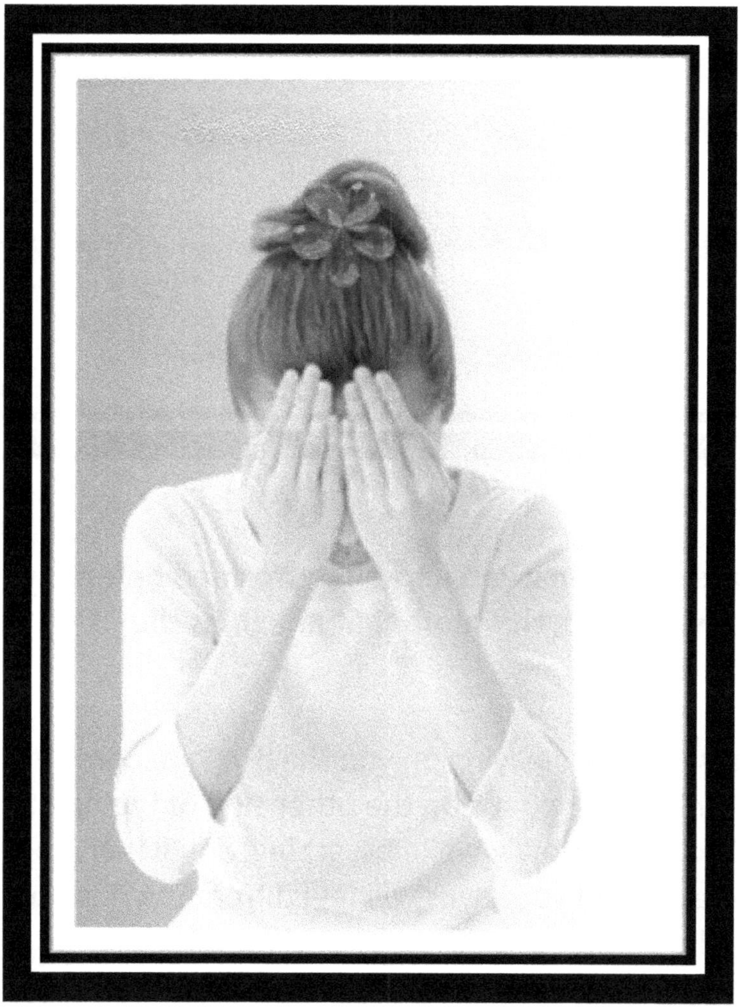

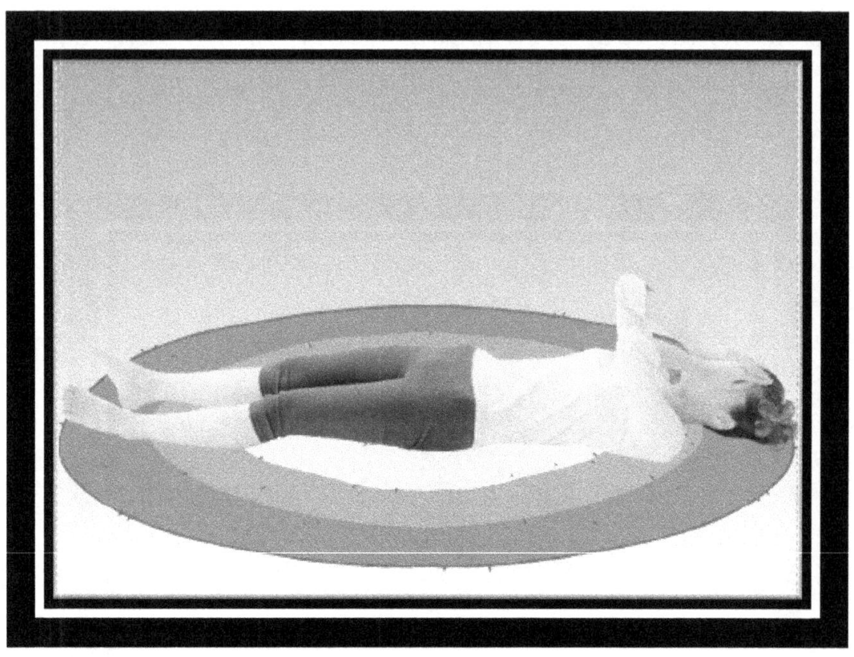

In the illumination method performed before going to bed, the room that imagines the universe is

It is done while lying on your back in a dark room. Think about what's on the other side of the night. If you do it slowly while breathing, you'll feel more relaxed and your eyes will feel different when you wake up the next day.

The six points of eye stimulation in eye yoga

The next way, called "six-point stimulation of the eyes," can help both eye problems and body distortions.

In fact, different parts of the body are linked to and related to the area around the eyes. The changes and problems that happen in the eyes are also signs that the body is out of shape.
The six points of eye stimulation in eye yoga

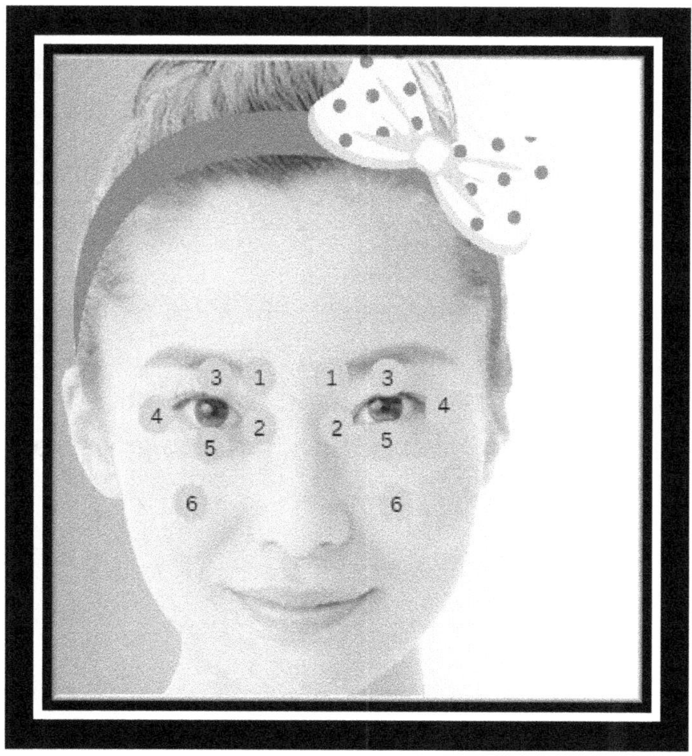

- No 1   Point   (between the eyebrows) Relieves eye fatigue caused by nervous tension
- No 2   Point   (inner eye) Eliminate eye fatigue caused by hand and arm fatigue
- No 3   Point   (above eye socket) Relieves eye fatigue caused by brain fatigue
- No 4   Point   (eye corner) Relieves eye fatigue caused by leg fatigue
- No 5   Point   (under the cheekbone) regulate intraocular pressure
- No 6   Point   (lower orbit) Eliminate eye fatigue caused by liver and gastrointestinal fatigue

When we try really hard to look at something, our eyebrows tend to tense up and get vertical lines.

Hold your eyebrows between your thumb and fingers, breathe in, and then breathe out as you rub. When you breathe out, you should picture bad energy leaving your mouth. I'm also going to take a stiff neck.

The second point , The hands and arms are connected to the inner area of the eye. When you use your hands and arms too much for computer work or chores, your eyes get tired.
computer work or chores, your eyes get tired.

There is an easy test that proves it. Raise both arms straight up in front of the mirror and compare the lengths of the left and right hands. When you raise your arms again, you'll see that your right hand goes up smoothly and your arm gets longer.

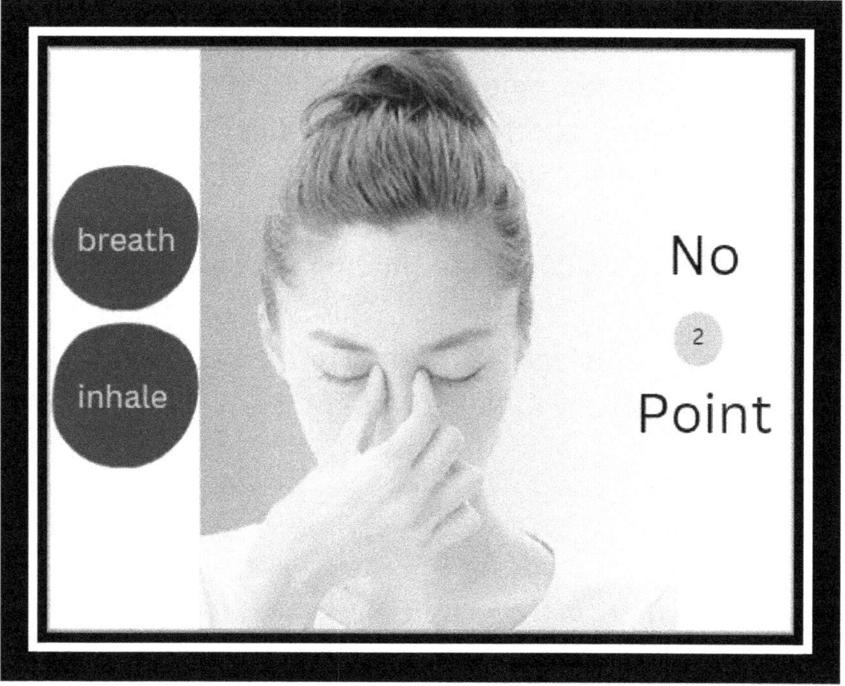

The third point is effective for eye fatigue caused by brain fatigue. In the beginning, the eye and the brain were linked by the optic nerve and had a strong connection. Place your thumb on the upper side of the edge of the bone around your eye. As you exhale, push up from the bottom to the top to ease brain fatigue and fix the imbalance between your left and right brain.

Change where your thumb is a little at a time to the left and right as you apply pressure. Pay attention to the areas that feel like they are working. You should be able to tell that your field of view is wider and brighter.

The fourth point , the outer corner of the eye, is closely related to the legs. If the blood flow to your legs isn't good or if your left and right legs aren't balanced, your eyes will get tired.

Press the outside part of the bone at the corner of the eye as you breathe out. This not only helps your eyes and legs feel better, but it also fixes any problems with your left and right legs.

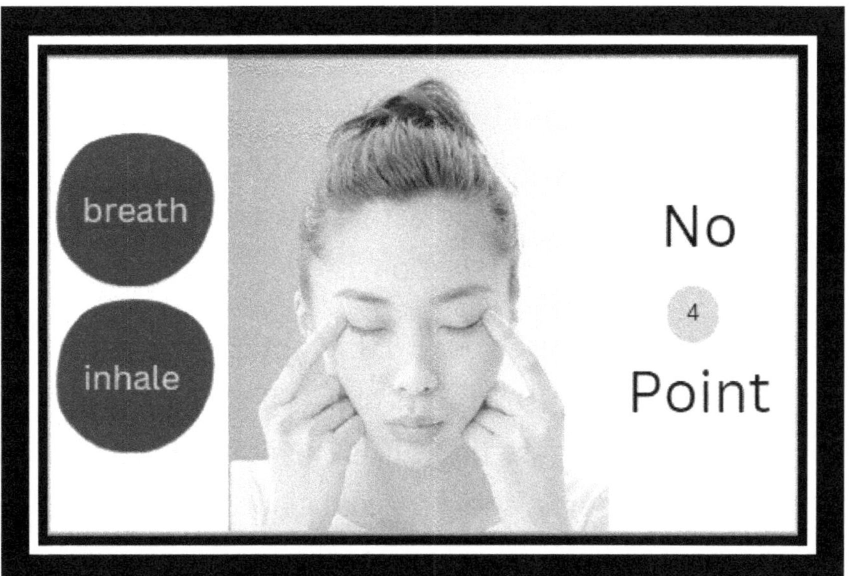

The fifth point , under the orbit, is when the liver and stomach are tired, fatigue accumulates under the eyes, and sagging and dark circles are likely to occur.

Place your index finger under the rim of the eyebone and press downward while exhaling. There is also a work to balance the internal organs such as liver and stomach.

Before and after shiatsu, try pressing around the bottom of the ribs and check for changes in hardness and pain. If you stimulate the side that feels hardness and pain more, it will be more effective.

The sixth point , below the cheekbone, is recommended for those with elevated intraocular pressure and eye congestion.

When eye pressure goes up, the optic nerve gets damaged and crushed. This makes it easier to get glaucoma, a disease that hurts the optic nerve and makes it harder to see. To avoid glaucoma, push up from the bottom of the cheekbone with your middle finger.

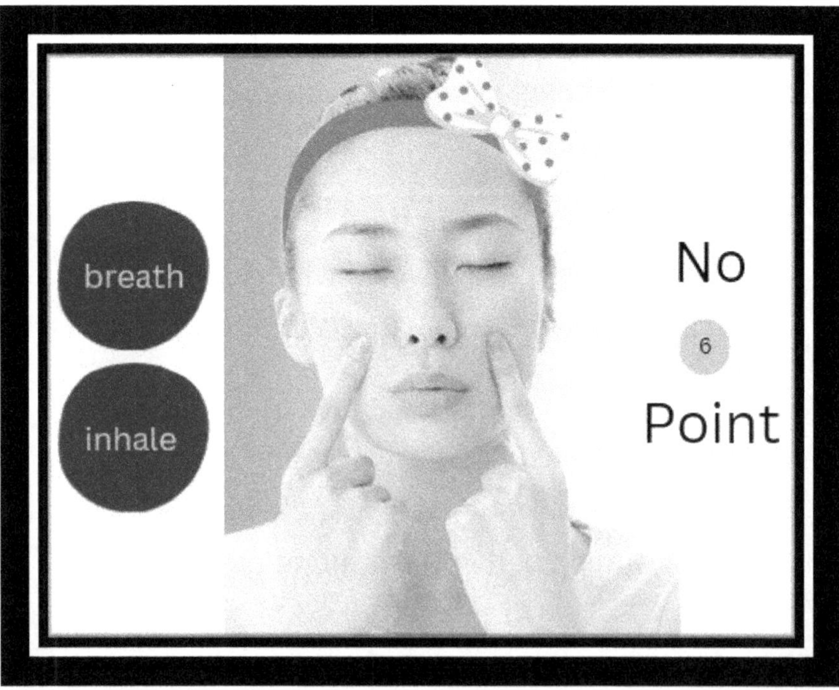

"Six-point stimulation" isn't just exciting; it's also important to make sure that your breathing and mind (image) are in sync. Think of "bad energy" leaving your mouth as you exhale to give yourself a boost. In just 2–3 minutes, you should feel like your eyes are no longer tired.

Eliminate lack of eye exercise! Improved body flexibility!

In this part, we'll talk about exercises for your eyes and arms that you can easily do at your office desk.

If you use a computer or smartphone for a long time and stare at the same screen, your eye movements will slow down and your eye muscles won't get enough work.

Just like your arm muscles get stiff if you don't move them, your eye muscles get stiff if you stare at your phone or computer screen for too long. Eye muscles that have been used too much and become hard have poor blood flow and store substances that make you tired. So, it's important to move the eyeballs along with the rest of the body when stretching. This will help relax the eye muscles and get more blood to the eyes.

If the blood flow around the eyes is improved, waste products and substances that make you tired will be flushed out, the eye muscles will become more flexible, and the eyes' natural abilities will be brought back. By combining the movements of the arm and the eye, "arm stretch and eye exercise" can move the eye a lot and loosen up tight eye muscles.

Also, moving both arms a lot loosens up stiffness in the neck, shoulders, and back, improves blood flow, and gets rid of tiredness.

Especially with the eyes, it's a good idea to move them so big that it seems like too much. Along with moving your arms, try to move your eyes as much as possible up and down.

How to use eye yoga to do "arm stretches and eye exercises."

Put your hands together in front of your chest (gassho) and straighten your back. Raise your hands up to relax tension in your shoulders and back.

Straighten your back, put your palms together, and adjust your breathing.

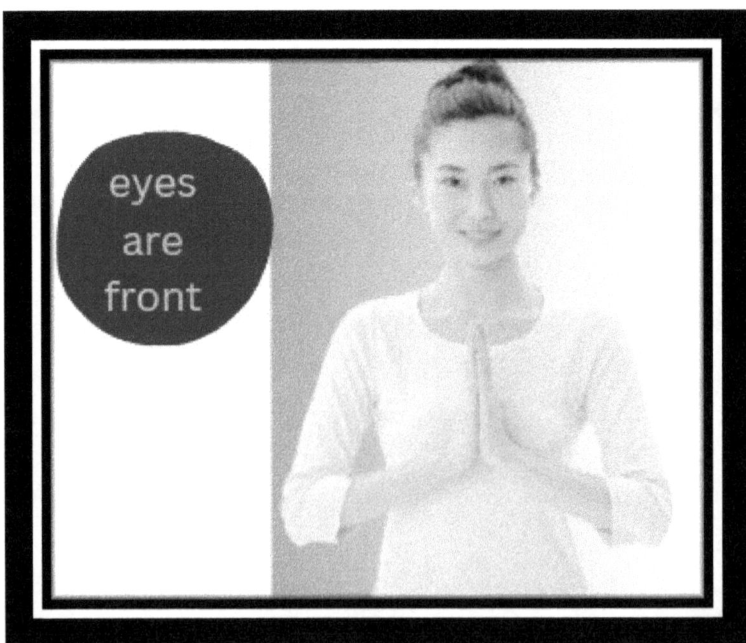

2   While breathing in, stretch your palms together high above your head. Extend as high as possible. At this time, look up while following your fingertips with your eyes. Don't move your face, just move your eyes.

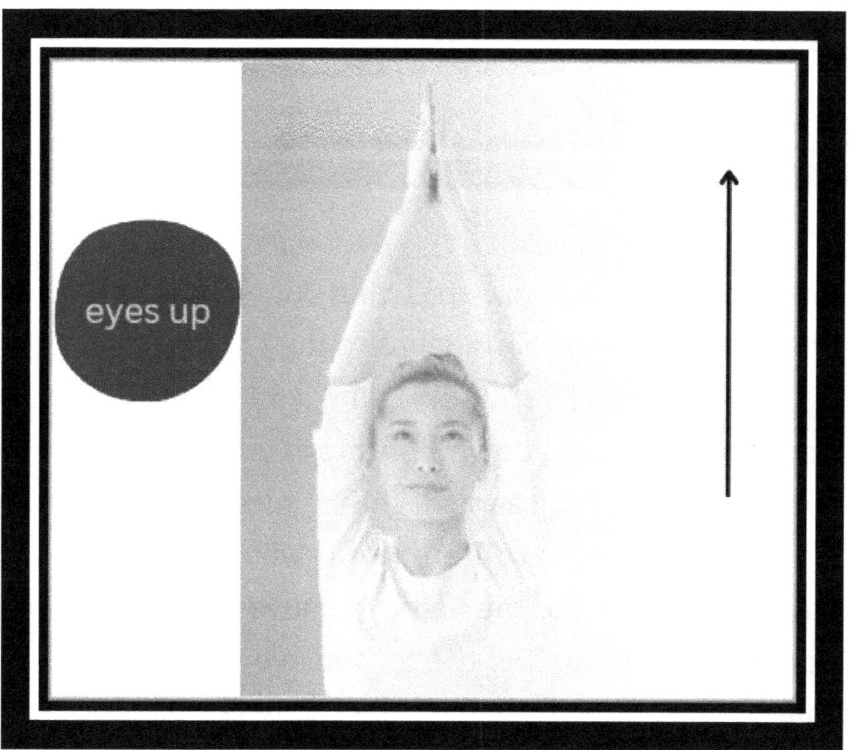

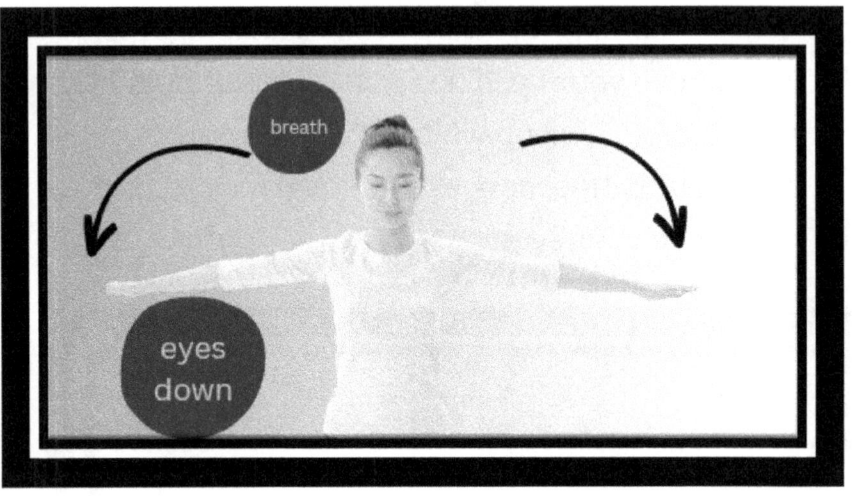

3. Once your arms are fully stretched out, let out a breath as you lower your palms to the left and right, hands facing out. At this time, you should also move your eyes down. Just move your eyes, not your face. If you can do it three times, try moving your eyes in a different way when you put down your hand. For the first eye, move vertically from top to bottom. For the second eye, look at your right hand and go down clockwise. For the third eye, look at your left hand and go down anticlockwise.

Once your arms are fully stretched out, let out a breath as you lower your palms to the left and right, hands facing out. At this time, you should also move your eyes down. Just move your eyes, not your face.

4. Finally put your hands together and adjust your breathing.

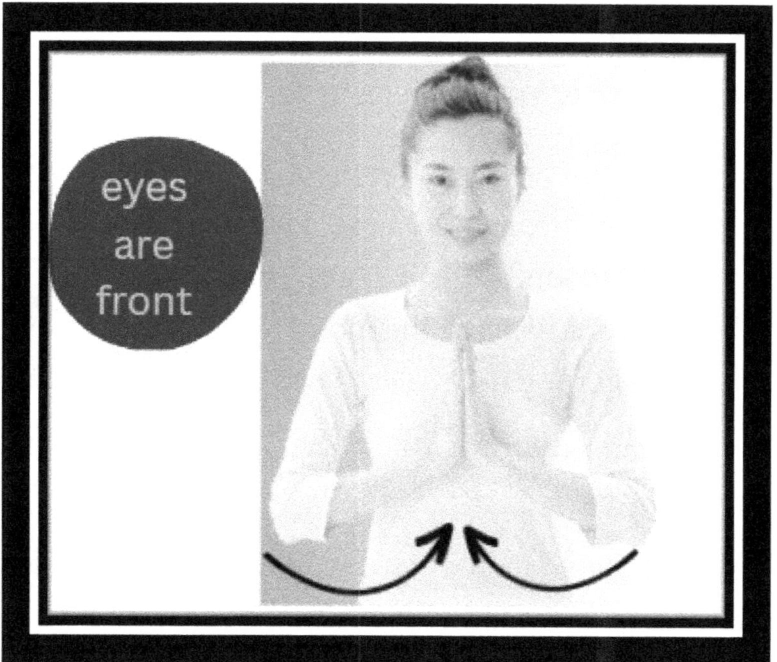

Breathe deeply and get oxygen to your eyes

If you use your eyes too much while working on your phone or computer, your breathing will get short, which is also a problem. This is because oxygen is important for the visual nerve to work well.

So do yoga cleansing breathing and switch from shallow to deep breathing to get air to your eyes.

Yoga's method for purifying the breath is to slowly breathe in through the nose, imagining that you are getting lots of fresh energy, and slowly breathe out through the mouth, imagining that you are getting rid of all the bad energy and waste products. By taking these deep breaths over and over, your mind and body will start to feel calmer.

As was stated in another section, it's important for the body and mind to move at the same time (image).

When you breathe in through your nose, stretch your arms and think that you are taking in a lot of new energy.

When you breathe out through your mouth, lower your arms and picture bad energy and waste products leaving your body. If you keep doing this, your whole body, your breathing, and your mind will move as one, and the effect of eye yoga will be even stronger.

Therapeutic yoga techniques include exercises such as

1. Palming
2. Blinking
3. Eyes moving side to side in simultaneous focus
4. Eyes turned sideways and forward at the same time
5. Rotational viewing
6. Viewing upwards and down simultaneously
7. Preliminary nose tip gazing
8. Near and distant viewing

1. Palming

- Close your eyes, sit still, and take some deep breaths to fully unwind.
- Rub your palms together hard until they get warm, then place them softly on your eyelids.
- Feel the warmth of your hands move to your eyes and relax your eye muscles. Your eyes are being bathed in dark, which feels good.
- Stay in this position until the eyes have fully absorbed the heat from your hands.
- Make sure your eyes are closed and your hands are not in your face. Rub the hands together again, and do this at least three more times.

2. Blinking

- Relax and keep your eyes open.
- Quickly blink around 10 times.
- Close your eyes and take 20 seconds to calm down. Slowly focus on how you're breathing.
- About 5 times, do this workout.

3. Eyes moving side to side in simultaneous focus

- Sit down with your legs straight out in front of you.
- Now, lift your arms while keeping your fists closed and pointing your hands up.
- Look at something straight in front of you at eye level.
- Keep your head in this position and look at the following one after the other by moving your eyes.
- The area between the eyes
- Right thumb
- The area between the eyes
- Right finger
- The area between the eyes
- Right thumb
- Ten to twenty times, do this practise.
- Close your eyes and take a break when you're done with this exercise.
- When you do the above practise, pay attention to how you breathe.
- Inhale while in the middle position.
- Look to the side as you let out your breath.
- Take a breath in and come back to the middle.

4. Eyes turned sideways and forward at the same time

- Straighten your legs and sit down.
- Then, put the left (closed) hand on the left knee with the thumb facing up.
- Look at something straight in front of you and at eye level.
- Having the head stay in this position.
- As you let your breath out, keep your eyes on your left thumb.
- As you take a deep breath in, look at something straight in front of you.
- Do the same thing again with your right thumb.
- Then shut your eyes and take a break.

5. Rotational viewing

- Keeping your legs straight in front of you, sit down.
- Put the left hand on the knee on the left side.
- Hold your right hand above your right knee with your thumb facing up. Don't bend your arm.
- Now, keep your head still and look at your thumb.
- Keep the arm straight and make a circle with the thumb.
- Do this exercise five times going both clockwise and anticlockwise.
- Repeat the process with your left thumb.

- Close your eyes, rest them, and let go of everything.
- During this exercise, you should breathe in the following way:
- As you make the top arc of the circle, breathe in.

- As you finish the lower circle, let out your breath.

6. Viewing upwards and down simultaneously

- Keeping your legs straight in front of you, sit down.
- Place both hands on your knees with your thumbs pointing up.
- Raise your right thumb slowly while keeping your arms straight. Follow the thumb as it moves up with your eyes.
- When the thumb is as high as it can go, slowly lower it back to the starting position while keeping your eyes on the thumb and your head still.
- Do the same thing again with your left thumb.
- This should be done five times with each thumb.
- Head and neck should stay straight the whole time.

- Close your eyes and take it easy.

- When you do the above practise, pay attention to how you breathe.

- Inhale as you raise your eyes.

- Exhale as you close your eyes.

7. **Preliminary nose tip gazing**

- Sit with your legs crossed.
- Straighten the right arm out in front of the nose.
- With your right hand, make a fist and keep your thumb pointing up.
- Focus both eyes on the end of the thumb.
- Now, bend your arm and slowly bring your thumb to the tip of your nose while keeping your eyes on the tip of your thumb.
- Stay in this pose for a while, holding your thumb at the tip of your nose and focusing your eyes there.

- Keeping your eyes on the tip of your thumb, slowly straighten your arm.

- The first round is over.
- Do at least five rounds like this.

- When you do the above practise, pay attention to how you breathe.

- Take a breath in while pulling the thumb to the tip of the nose.

- Hold the thumb at the tip of the nose and stay inside.

- As the arm goes straight, let out your breath.

8. Near and distant viewing

- Stand or sit by a window that lets you see the sky clearly. Keep your arms next to you.
- For 5–10 seconds, look at the tip of the nose.
- Do this about ten to twenty times.
- Close your eyes and take a break.
- Notice the following way of breathing
- When looking up close, take a breath.
- When looking far away, let out a breath.

Here is a series of remedies to help the eyes not be tired and sore .

- Vitamin A and lutein are both good for your eyes and help them feel better. Here is a list of things that have them:

- Vitamin A and lutein can be found in carrots, spinach, and kale.

- lutein is found in zucchini, chard and Brussels sprouts;

- Vitamin A comes from sweet potatoes and butter; Be careful with butter, it's good for the eyes but bad for your health.

- liver (which is high in vitamin A), such as cod liver oil;

Herbal remedies to improve eyesight

Here are some of the herbs beneficial for eye health :

- Chamomile is a decongestant and moisturiser. Blueberries improve vision and are used to treat eye problems and cataracts.
- mallow is soothing and moisturising, and it helps keep the eyes moist. It is great for people who are sensitive to light and for people who usually wear contact lenses.
- Ginkgo Biloba is an antioxidant that improves blood flow and is used to treat glaucoma and visual degeneration.
- Calendula is an anti-inflammatory plant that is often used in eye drops to make them feel better.

Other natural remedies for better eyesight

In addition to what is written, we also remember other good practices that can relieve eye fatigue :

- pour cold water into your open eyes;
- Palming, which is when you rub your hands together to warm them up and place them over your eyes without touching them for about ten breaths;
- If you spend a lot of time in front of a screen, it's good for you to look away from time to time.

55

- Think of these workouts as a chance to take a break and do something for yourself.Find a place to sit where you can be relaxed and keep your back straight.
- As with yoga, the prize comes from being consistent. If you could find a few minutes every day, the benefits would be clear right away.
- Important: You can't do yoga eye movements if you're wearing glasses or contacts.

Advice for healthy eyes

1.Reduce your time spent in front of displays (computers, smartphones, and televisions) because they can cause eye strain and decrease your vision. If you are unable to reduce your screen time, use eye drops and close your eyes for 20 seconds every 20 minutes to allow them to relax.

2. In bright sunlight, wear sunglasses with 100% UV protection. Keep a pair in your bag at all times.

3. Avoid smoking because it is harmful to your eyes.

Consume a well-balanced diet rich in fresh vegetables and fruits, "good" fats, and whole grains.

5. Exercise on a daily basis to help maintain a healthy BMI, which aids in the prevention of heart disease and diabetes.

6. Schedule frequent eye checkups with an eye doctor who can spot the earliest signs of any eye ailment or disease.

7. Aim for 7 to 9 hours of sleep per night.

8. Maintain proper hygiene and wash your hands frequently if you rub or contact your eyes to avoid infection.

9. Use high-quality lighting, such as LEDs that resemble natural light, to keep your eyes comfortable.

10. Perform a few minutes of easy yet strong yoga eye exercises every day.

Tips to reduce eye strain

As has already been said, too much time spent in front of computers is the main cause of eye strain. The best advice we could give you is to spend as much time as possible outside and away from your phone. But we know that this isn't always possible, so we suggest that you give yourself some room. It doesn't take much: every now and then, look away, look out the window, and give yourself a break.

In short, even if you have to think about something else, take care of yourself.

A letter of emotion that arrived at "Eye Yoga"

As was said above, the main reason why people's eyes are tired and their vision is getting worse is because they use their phones and computers too much.

In particular, there is no limit to the number of people whose eyesight has suddenly gotten worse after they switched from a regular cell phone to a smartphone.

The other day, a 24-year-old woman who had read my Eye Yoga book sent me a letter that made me feel good. The woman said that her eyesight had never been bad, even when she was young, and that she always got an A, which is the best score on an eyesight test.

But when he went to college and got a smartphone instead of a flip phone, he started using communication apps (like LINE) and games, and the amount of time he spent looking at his phone quickly grew to the point where he became hooked to it.

Even though I should have been able to see well, I soon had trouble seeing things in the distance.

When I look around, I see that all of my friends have bad eyesight and wear glasses or contact lenses. He thought that if he kept doing this, his eyesight would only get worse, so he decided to look for something that would be good for his eyes.

When she found eye yoga, she tried it right away. Her blurry eyes cleared up right away, and she could see things that were hard to see before. One reason why eye yoga is encouraged is because it works right away.

Please try to do the eye yoga we talked about this time every day. Not only will your eyes feel better, but also your body and mind will feel better.

The 12 Healthiest Foods for Your Eyes

Eat the best healthy foods for your eyes to keep your vision in good shape.

We already know that our bodies work best when they get whole, hearty foods. This is also true when it comes to certain parts of the body. Your eyes are a good example.

If you eat more of the best foods for eye health, you give your eyes what they need. In other words, if you want to make sure you can see well for the rest of your life, you should eat things that are good for your eyes. What are they then? We should find out.

Here are 12 foods that are good for your eyes, whether you have a history of vision problems in your family or are trying to avoid eye strain every day.

Broccoli is a vegetable.

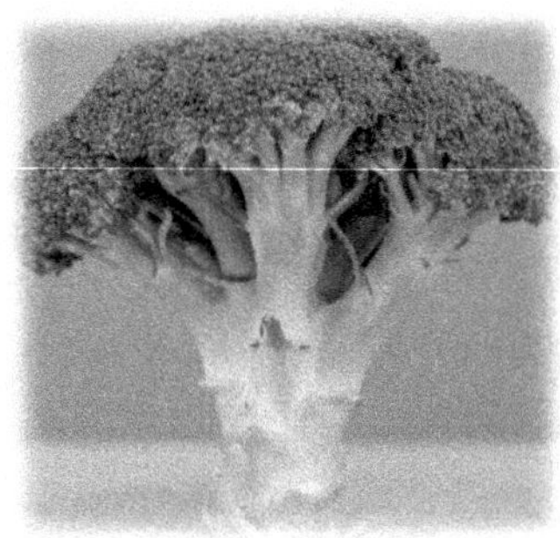

A study that was backed by the American Optometric Association found that a substance in broccoli called indole-3-carbinol can help get rid of toxins in your retina. This lowers your chance of getting age-related macular degeneration, which is one of the main reasons why older people lose their sight. Broccoli also has lutein and zeaxanthin, which are also good for your eyes because they protect them. But keep in mind that this study

says you would have to eat a lot of broccoli to
really protect yourself from AMD.

Salmon is a fish.

To keep your eyes healthy, you need to make sure they get enough water. Some of the best foods for good eyes can take you a long way. Omega-3 fatty acids are found in salmon, for example. This makes you less likely to get dry eyes, which is a painful condition that gets more common as you get older.

If you're a woman, it's more important for your eyes to eat fish and other foods with omega-3s. People who were born female are twice as likely to have dry eyes.

Carrots

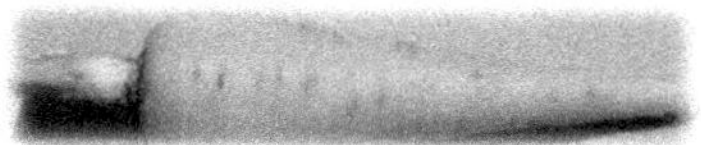

You've probably heard this before: carrots are one of the best things for your eyes. First of all, they have a lot of beta-carotene, which is an antioxidant your body uses to make vitamin A. Vitamin A helps you see at night and keeps your eyes from getting too nearsighted, which is called myopia. Grab Bugs Bunny's favorite snack if you want to avoid needing vision correction or keep your current prescription for contacts or eyeglasses as long as possible.

Plus, carrots have another antioxidant called lutein. This one can make you less likely to get AMD..

Sunflower grains

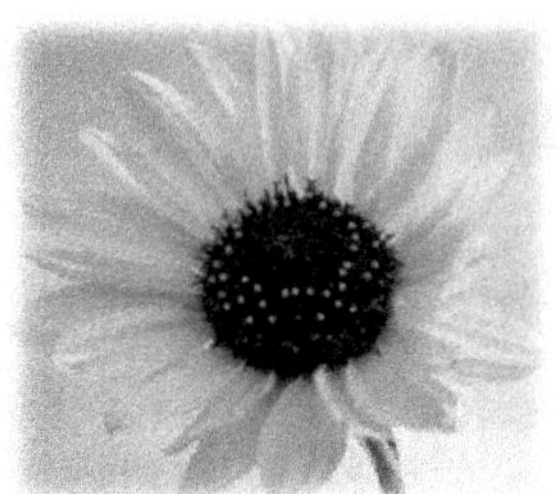

Yes, you should keep the sun out of your eyes. But don't be fooled by the name. There's no need for safety here. One of the best things for your eyes is sunflower seeds. They have a lot of vitamin E, which is an antioxidant that saves our eyes from damage caused by free radicals. Vitamin E also protects your eyes from the sun's harmful UV rays, which lowers your risk of getting cataracts.

One important thing to remember is that your body can make some vitamins, but it can't make vitamin E on its own. You have to get vitamin E from food or pills.

Kiwi

Want another way to protect yourself from possible sun damage? Kiwi can help. This fuzzy fruit is on our list of the best foods for healthy eyes because it has lutein, the vitamin that fights AMD, and zeaxanthin, which helps your eyes filter light.

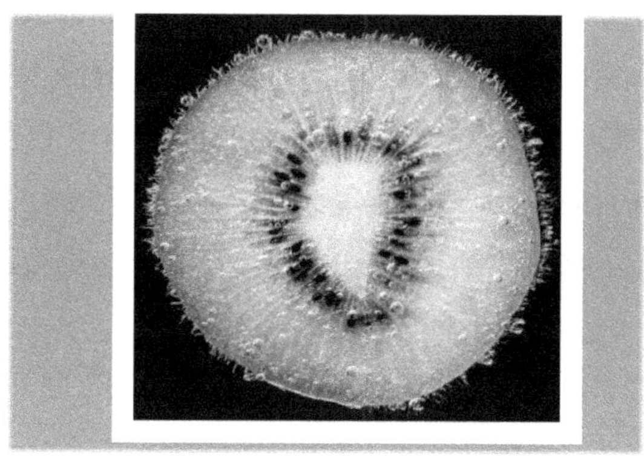

The shellfish oysters

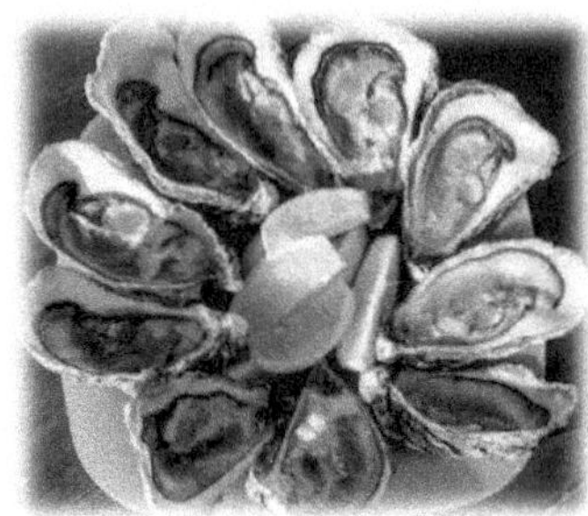

Some of the other things that are good for eye health might not have come as much of a surprise, but this one might. Even so, it's still worth it to get shucking. Oysters not only have omega-3 fatty acids, but they also have a lot of iron. This gives you a powerful nutrient that can help you fight AMD.

Spinach

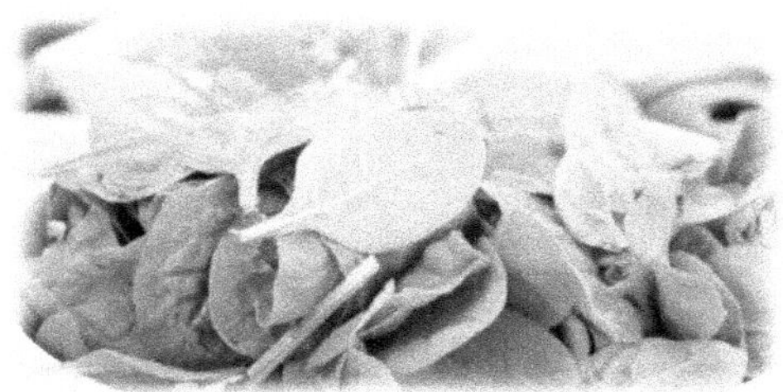

Think like Popeye and consume your spinach. This leafy green is one of the greatest foods for healthy eyes since it contains a wide variety of essential elements. As I've mentioned, lutein is essential to good eye health, and it's present in high concentrations here. Zeaxanthin can also be found in spinach.

Antioxidants are better absorbed by the body when eaten with fat. The best foods for eyesight can be easily incorporated into any meal by including a small spinach salad dressed with olive oil, which also contains omega-9s and a little quantity of omega-3s.

Eggs

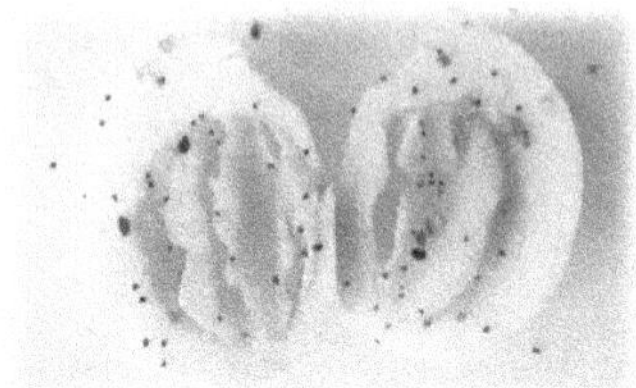

Eggs provide all the nutrients necessary for healthy eyes, including the antioxidants lutein and zeaxanthin, as well as zinc and vitamin A. In fact, a 2019 study found that eating eggs on a regular basis (about two to four eggs per week) greatly reduces the chance of developing AMD. Eggs are a convenient go-to option if you're looking to eat foods that support healthy eyes.

Almonds

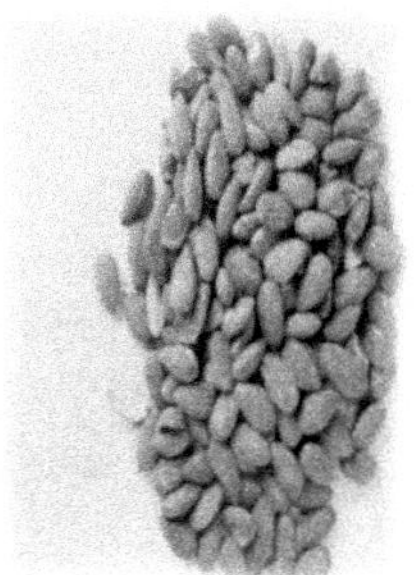

Vitamin E, an antioxidant that can help prevent macular degeneration and cataracts, is abundant in almonds and other nuts. Once again, this is a vitamin that your body simply doesn't produce.

In addition, if you're short on time, this is one of the best foods to improve your eyes' health. A handful of almonds can be eaten on the move without the need for a burner or chopping board.

Yogurt

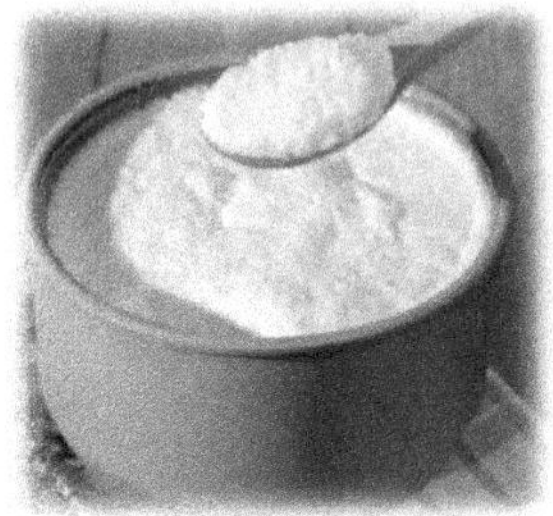

Vitamin A and zinc, two elements I've already mentioned as being essential for eye health, may be found in dairy products. However, cultured dairy products are the greatest option if you're trying to improve your eyesight through what you eat. Why? Because probiotics can be found in yogurt. More and more research suggests that these beneficial bacteria could alleviate a wide range of eye complaints, from allergic conjunctivitis to dry eye.

Oranges

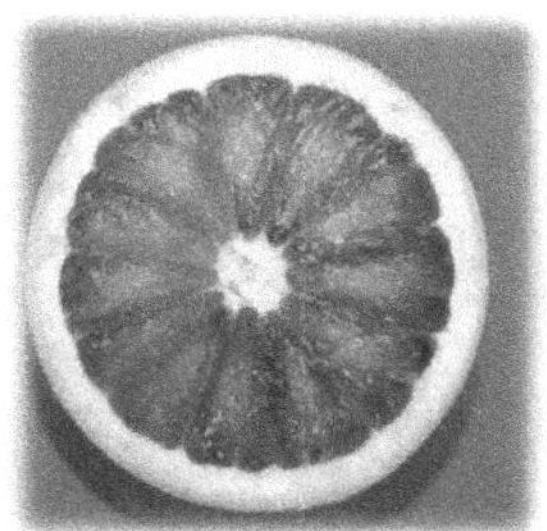

I've already explained how and why beta-carotene contributes to vitamin A, and why that's important for maintaining healthy eyes. What I didn't mention, though, is that beta-carotene-containing foods are readily available because of the color orange imparted by the antioxidant. Oranges, which are known to contain a sizable amount of this nutrient, are included here since they are among the finest foods for improving eye health.

Also, oranges are a good source of vitamin C, as you undoubtedly already know. And that can help your body battle age-related macular degeneration, cataracts, and vision loss altogether.

Strawberries

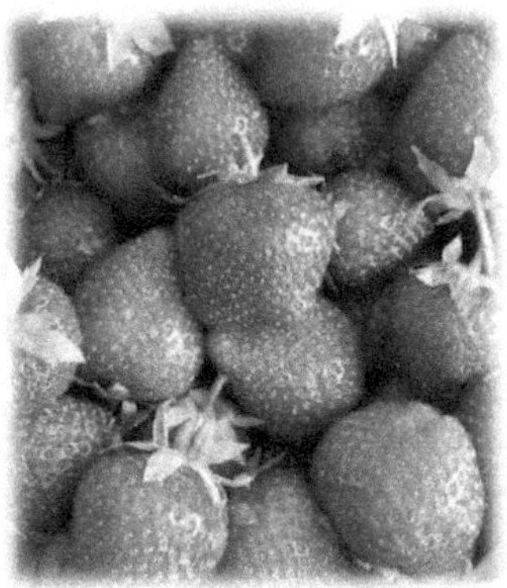

Although oranges get more press, strawberries really have higher levels of vitamin C. These berries should be included in our list of the finest foods for eye health because of the vitamin C they contain, which provides a one-two-three punch against macular degeneration, cataracts, and general vision loss.

What Are Yoga Eye Pillows?

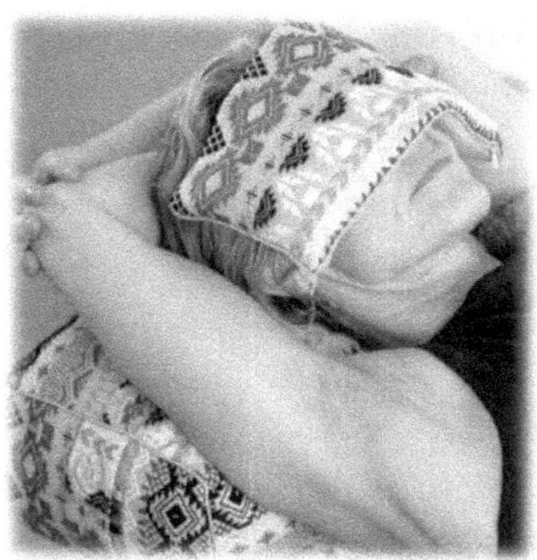

Small, weighted pillows that you can put over your eyes are called yoga eye pillows. They are small and rectangle, and one pillow can be used to cover both eyes.

There are many different colors and designs of yoga eye pillows, but the fabric should be soft. So, when you put the pillow over your eyes, you'll feel at ease.

Even if you don't do yoga very often, you should always have a pillow with you. So, you can get the benefits of them even if you don't do yoga.

How an eye pillow works

Yoga eye covers block out light and give your eyes a little bit of pressure. The pillow can also stimulate your vagus nerve, which is one of the nerves that connects your lungs, heart, and digestive system.

When you stimulate the vagus nerve, changes happen all over your body. These changes can help you feel calmer. From your neck to your pelvis, the vagus nerve controls many systems, so it can help you feel calm.

Blocking out the light with an eye pillow can also help you relax and fall asleep. If your room isn't completely dark, the pillow can make it darker. It will then be easier for you to fall asleep.

Uses for an Eye Pillow

A yoga eye pillow can be used at any time of the day or week. Of course, it's a great way to end a yoga lesson and relax. During savasana, you can use the pillow to help you stay in the moment and not look around the room.You don't have to practice yoga, though, to use a yoga eye pillow. You can also use one at night to help you fall asleep. The extra darkness and small pressure can make it easier for you to fall asleep, so you can sleep more.

When you feel worried or stressed, you can use the pillow. You can take advantage of the vagus nerve activation by lying down and putting a pillow over your eyes.

A lot of things, like deep breathing and meditation, can get the vagus nerve going. Even though the pressure on your eyes isn't enough on its own, the pillow can still help you relax. This can help you breathe deeply and focus.

Then, it can help you feel better by balancing your mood and feelings.

Try to pay attention to each part of your body or relax to get the most out of your eye pillow. Don't count too much on your pillow to make you feel calm.

Benefits of a Yoga Eye Pillow

If you want to use a yoga eye pillow, you should understand how it can help you. Here are a few great ways that an eye pillow can help you, whether you want to use it at the end of a yoga lesson or at the end of a long day.

Set rules for digestion

The first and probably most shocking way a yoga eye pillow can help you is by regulating your digestion. This is related to the vagus nerve, which is linked to your gut system. When you trigger the vagus nerve, you can make it easier for your body to break down food.

It might even help with some stomach problems, but you should talk to your doctor about your particular situation. Overall, though, the pressure from the pillow can help awaken the vagus nerve and improve digestion.You might not see a big change, and the word "change" has more than one meaning. But a yoga eye pillow can help with digestive problems along with other methods. It could help you digest the things you love better.

Slow your heartbeat

Your heart rate can also go down with the help of a yoga eye pillow. Again, this has to do with the vagus nerve, and a slower heart rate can help with a lot of things. You can use the pillow to slow down your heart rate if you have a fast heart rate normally or if your heart beats faster because of stress.

When you fall asleep, your heart rate also slows down a bit. This helps you save energy and completely unwind. But if you can't get to sleep, you might need help getting your heart rate down.

Even though a yoga eye pillow can't replace medical care, it might help. But there is also a chance that you will slow your heart rate too much. If you already have a lower-than-average heart rate, you might not want to use a yoga eye pillow.

Don't let light in

Make your room as dark as possible if you need help going asleep. But roommates, clocks, and other things that give off light can make that hard to do. You can block light with many things, like eye masks or eye pillows.

A yoga eye pillow can block out light, and the small pressure can help you close your eyes. Then you won't have to worry as much that too much light will make it hard for you to sleep.

You can instead enjoy the dark room and how the eye pillow makes you feel calm. Now, if you move around a lot while you sleep, an eye pillow might not be the best thing for you. But if you don't move and sleep on your back, it may be the perfect answer.

Change your mood

Your vagus nerve also goes to your brain, and if you can control that nerve, you can change how you feel. Using an eye pillow might help if you've been feeling stressed or worried. Putting the pillow on your eyes for a few minutes might make you feel better.

Like the other perks, a yoga eye pillow is not a replacement for medical care. If you have depression or worry, you might want to think about going to a therapist. But an eye pillow can be a great way to treat small mood changes at home.

It's a good reason to lie down for a while. Take a break from work or chores around the house and have some fun. You can use the pillow whenever you want to make yourself feel better.

Keeping the nervous system in check

Using a yoga eye pillow can also help keep your nerve system in balance. When you stimulate the vagus nerve, it can send messages throughout your body that make you feel good. You don't need to be upset or have stomach problems to use the pillow.

The pressure from the pillow can affect your whole body, whether you use it for yoga or something else. The pressure can make you feel good, so even though it seems strange at first, you may come to like using the pillow.Even though the pillow won't treat or fix diseases of the nervous system, you should try it. It can be used in addition to surgery or regular medicines. Then you can get the most out of the treatments you have.

One Last Thing

Yoga eye pillows are small pillows that you put over your eyes, but you don't have to use them during a yoga lesson. They can help your brain and body in many ways, so you should try one. You never know when you'll need it.

www.ingramcontent.com/pod-product-compliance
Lightning Source LLC
Chambersburg PA
CBHW071610270726
48661CB00019B/2023